Dash Diet Recipes

-A Beginner's Cookbook with Low Sodium Recipes to Lose Weight Permanently and Live Healthy-

[Sebastian Osborne]

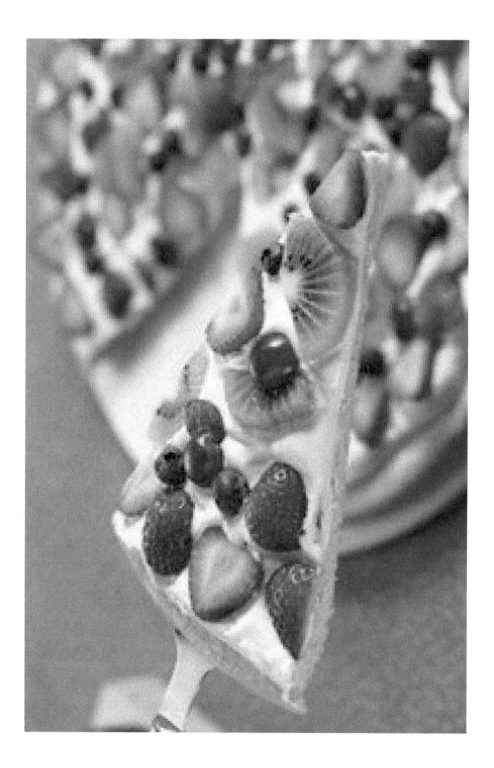

Table Of Content

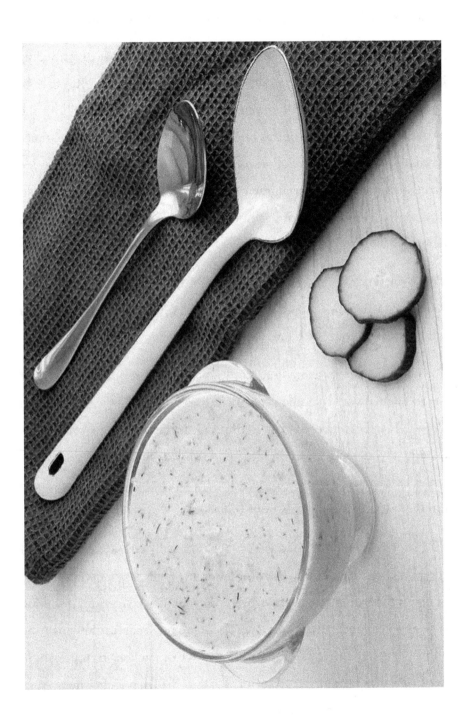

The following Book is reproduced below with the goal of providing information that is as accurate and reliable as possible. Regardless, purchasing this Book can be seen as consent to the fact that both the publisher and the author of this book are in no way experts on the topics discussed within and that any recommendations or suggestions that are made herein are for entertainment purposes only. Professionals should be consulted as needed prior to undertaking any of the action endorsed herein.

This declaration is deemed fair and valid by both the American Bar Association and the Committee of Publishers Association and is legally binding throughout the United States.

Furthermore, the transmission, duplication, or reproduction of any of the following work including specific information will be considered an illegal act irrespective of if it is done electronically or in print. This extends to creating a secondary or tertiary copy of the work or a recorded copy and is only allowed with the express written consent from the Publisher. All additional right reserved.

The information in the following pages is broadly considered a truthful and accurate account of facts and as such, any inattention, use, or misuse of the information in question by the reader will render any resulting actions solely under their purview. There are no scenarios in which the publisher or the original author of this work can be in any fashion deemed liable for any hardship or damages that may befall them after undertaking information described herein.

Additionally, the information in the following pages is intended only for informational purposes and should thus be thought of as universal. As befitting its nature, it is presented without assurance regarding its prolonged validity or interim quality. Trademarks that are mentioned are done without written consent and can in no way be considered an endorsement from the trademark holder.

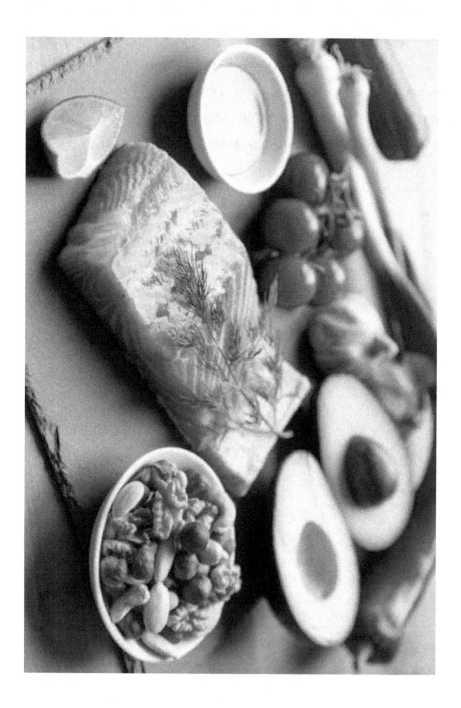

CHAPTER 1: **BREAKFAST**

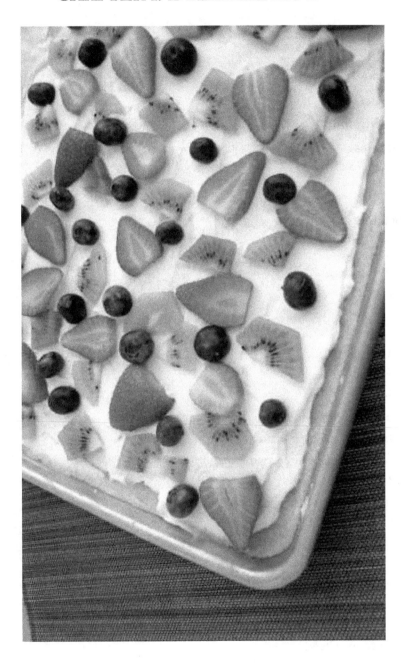

Fruit Pizza

Prep:

15 mins

Cook:

5 mins

Additional:

30 mins

Total:

50 mins

Servings:

8

Yield:

8 servings

Ingredients

Crust:

1 cup crushed cornflakes

2 tablespoons light corn syrup

2 tablespoons white sugar

2 tablespoons butter, softened

1 tablespoon honey

Frosting:

2 (8 ounce) packages cream cheese, softened

1 (7 ounce) jar marshmallow fluff

Toppings:

½ cup sliced strawberries

2 kiwi, peeled and sliced

2 apricots, sliced

Directions

1

Preheat oven to 350 degrees F.

2

Mix cornflakes, butter, corn syrup, and sugar in a bowl until evenly combined; press onto a baking sheet.

3

Bake in the preheated oven until crust is golden brown, about 5 minutes. Drizzle crust with honey and cool in refrigerator, about 15-17 minutes.

4

Stir cream cheese and marshmallow fluff together in a bowl until smooth and creamy; spread over cooled crust, keeping a 1/2-inch border of crust. Chill crust in refrigerator until completely cooled, about 15 minutes.

5

Arrange strawberries, apricots, and kiwi over the cream cheese layer.

Nutrition

Per Serving: 366 calories; protein 5.1g; carbohydrates 37.6g; fat 22.7g; cholesterol 69.2mg; sodium 235.1mg.

Warmed Stuffed Peaches

Prep:

20 mins

Cook:

10 mins

Additional:

8 hrs

Total:

8 hrs 30 mins

Servings:

4

Yield:

4 servings

Ingredients

Dressing:
1 medium red bell pepper, chopped
½ teaspoon garlic paste
¼ cup chopped yellow onion
2 tablespoons vegetable oil
2 tablespoons honey
¼ cup apple cider vinegar
½ teaspoon freshly grated ginger
Salad:
1 tablespoon vegetable oil
½ pound kale leaves, veins removed
⅓ cup goat cheese
2 peaches, each cut into 8 wedges
salt and pepper to taste

Directions

1

Combine red bell pepper, vinegar, onion, oil, honey, ginger, and garlic paste in a jar with a lid. Cover jar, shake, and refrigerate dressing 8 hours to overnight.

2

Preheat an outdoor grill for medium-high heat and lightly oil the grate.

3

Place peaches and kale on the preheated grill. Toss kale continuously until softened and lightly charred on the edges, about 5 minutes. Cook and turn peaches until grill marks appear, about 3 minutes per side.

4

Place cooked kale in a serving bowl and toss with dressing. Top with cooked peaches and goat cheese. Season with salt and pepper. Serve warm.

Nutrition

Per Serving: 223 calories; protein 4.8g; carbohydrates 20.5g; fat 14.2g; cholesterol 9.2mg; sodium 149.3mg.

Maple Oatmeal

Prep:

5 mins

Cook:

6 mins

Additional:

2 mins

Total:

13 mins

Servings:

1

Yield:

1 serving

Ingredients

1 ½ cups water

1 tablespoon maple syrup

1 tablespoon packed dark brown sugar

¾ cup quick-cooking oats

Directions

1

Bring water to a boil. Add oats and cook, stirring, for 1 minute. Remove from heat and stir in brown sugar and maple syrup. Let sit until desired thickness is reached, 2 to 4 minutes.

Nutrition

Per Serving: 334 calories; protein 8g; carbohydrates 67.9g; fat 4g; sodium 19.9mg.

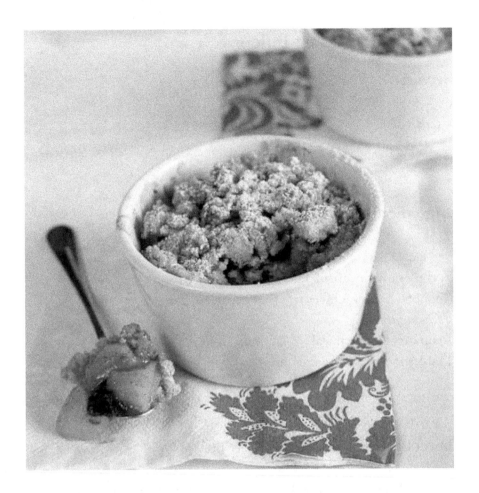

Creamy Breakfast Polenta

Servings:

6

Yield:

6 servings

Ingredients

3 ½ cups Silk® Unsweetened Coconutmilk
¼ cup non-dairy cream cheese
Chopped parsley, chives or other herbs, for garnish
1 teaspoon salt
1 cup organic cornmeal
1 tablespoon vegan margarine

Directions

1

Bring Silk and salt to a boil in a medium saucepan. Slowly stir in cornmeal.

2

Return to a boil, then reduce to a simmer and cook for 15 minutes until very thick, stirring often to prevent polenta from sticking to pan.

3

Remove from heat and stir in cream cheese and margarine until fully incorporated.

4

Spoon into a serving dish or press gently into a large oiled bowl, then turn over for molded polenta.

5

Garnish with parsley, chives or other chopped herbs.

Nutrition

Per Serving: 148 calories; protein 2g; carbohydrates 19g; fat 6.5g; sodium 479.5mg.

Banana Smoothie

Prep:

5 mins

Total:

5 mins

Servings:

1

Yield:

1 servings

Ingredients

1 cup milk

5 (1 gram) packets low calorie granulated sugar substitute (such as Sweet 'n Low®)

1 ½ bananas

Directions

1

Blend milk, bananas, and sugar substitute in a blender or food processor until smooth.

Nutrition

Per Serving: 280 calories; protein 10g; carbohydrates 56.8g; fat 5.4g; cholesterol 19.5mg; sodium 101.8mg.

Papaya Bruschetta

Prep:

20 mins

Total:

20 mins

Servings:

8

Yield:

8 servings

Ingredients

1 papaya
5 roma (plum) tomatoes, diced
¼ cup chopped fresh basil leaves
2 tablespoons white sugar
¼ cup red wine vinegar
½ red onion, diced
1 red bell pepper, seeded and diced
¼ cup vegetable oil
2 green onions, chopped
1 French baguette, cut into 1/2 inch pieces
½ teaspoon mustard powder

Directions

1

Cut papaya in half and remove seeds. Reserve 2 tablespoons of seeds for the dressing. Peel and dice the papaya, and place in a medium bowl. Add tomatoes, red onion, red pepper and basil, and set aside.

2

In a food processor or blender, combine the papaya seeds, sugar, wine vinegar, oil, mustard and green onions. Process until smooth and thick, and most of the seeds have broken up. Pour over the papaya mixture and stir to coat all of the ingredients. Serve with slices of baguette.

Nutrition

Per Serving: 263 calories; protein 7.5g; carbohydrates 41.1g; fat 8.1g; sodium 372.9mg.

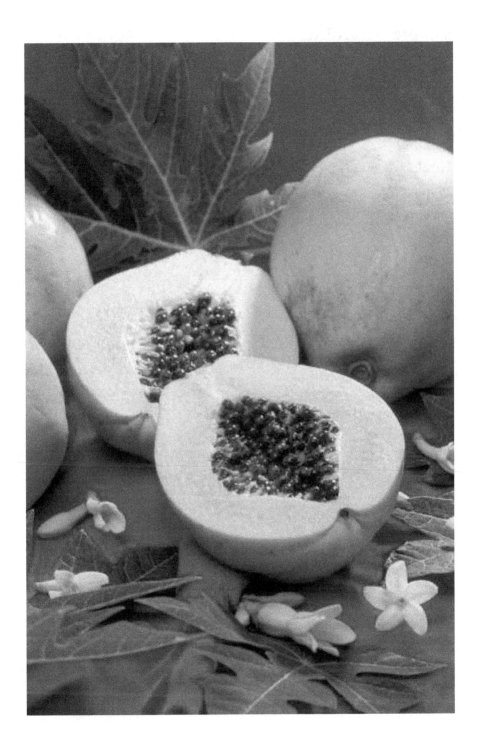

Veggie Scramble

Prep:

10 mins

Cook:

15 mins

Total:

25 mins

Servings:

6

Yield:

6 servings

Ingredients

¼ cup olive oil

¼ cup chopped onions

¼ cup chopped green bell peppers

¼ cup sliced fresh mushrooms

6 eggs

¼ cup chopped fresh tomato

¼ cup shredded Cheddar cheese

¼ cup milk

Directions

1

Heat olive oil in a skillet or frying pan over medium-high heat. Add mushrooms, onions and peppers; saute until onions are transparent.

2

In a mixing bowl, beat together eggs and milk. Add egg mixture to vegetables; stir in tomatoes. Cook until eggs are set. When eggs are almost done, mix in cheese. Serve immediately.

Nutrition

Per Serving: 182 calories; protein 8.1g; carbohydrates 2.4g; fat 15.8g; cholesterol 191.8mg; sodium 159.1mg.

Zucchini Waffles

15 mins

Cook:

5 mins

Total:

20 mins

Servings:

8

Yield:

8 waffles

Ingredients

2 eggs

1 tablespoon vegetable oil

1 pinch salt

½ cup dry potato flakes

¼ teaspoon onion powder

¼ teaspoon baking powder

3 cups shredded zucchini

Directions

1

Preheat a waffle iron according to manufacturer's instructions.

2

Mix zucchini, eggs, vegetable oil, onion powder, and salt together in a bowl. Stir in potato flakes and baking powder; mix until batter is combined.

3

Pour 1/2 cup of the batter onto the center of the waffle iron. Close the lid; cook until iron stops steaming and waffle is crisp, about 5 minutes.

Nutrition

Per Serving: 51 calories; protein 2.4g; carbohydrates 4.2g; fat 3g; cholesterol 46.5mg; sodium 59.9mg.

Chocolate Quinoa Cakes

Prep:

15 mins

Cook:

40 mins

Additional:

30 mins

Total:

1 hr 25 mins

Servings:

12

Yield:

12 servings

Ingredients

2 cups cold cooked quinoa

1 ¼ cups white sugar

¾ cup melted butter

4 eggs

⅓ cup milk

1 ½ teaspoons vanilla extract

1 cup cocoa powder

1 teaspoon baking soda

½ teaspoon salt

½ cup chocolate chips

1 ½ teaspoons baking powder

Directions

1

Preheat oven to 350 degrees F. Grease a rectangular cake pan.

2

Blend quinoa, butter, eggs, milk, and vanilla extract together in a blender until smooth.

3

Combine sugar, cocoa powder, baking powder, baking soda, and salt together in a large bowl. Stir quinoa mixture into sugar mixture until batter is well combined. Fold chocolate chips and pecans into batter; pour into the prepared pan.

4

Bake in the preheated oven until a toothpick inserted in the center of the cake comes out clean, 40 to 45 minutes. Cool cake on a wire rack.

Nutrition

Per Serving: 332 calories; protein 5.8g; carbohydrates 37g; fat 20.5g; cholesterol 93mg; sodium 374.9mg

Salsa Eggs

Prep:

30 mins

Total:

30 mins

Servings:

12

Yield:

12 servings

Ingredients

Eggs:
6 Eggland's Best Eggs, hard cooked and peeled
1 tablespoon sour cream
3 tablespoons fresh salsa or chunky salsa, drained, if necessary
Topping:
1 teaspoon Chopped fresh cilantro
2 teaspoons fresh salsa

Directions

1

Cut eggs in half lengthwise. Remove egg yolks; place yolks into bowl.

2

Mash yolks with fork. Add 3 tablespoons salsa and sour cream; mix well.

3

Spoon about 1 tablespoon egg yolk mixture into each egg white half.

4

Top each with about 1/2 teaspoon salsa and garnish with cilantro, if desired.

5

Cover and refrigerate until serving time or up to 24 hours.

Nutrition

Per Serving: 35 calories; protein 2.9g; carbohydrates 0.5g; fat 2.4g; cholesterol 93.6mg; sodium 61.1mg.

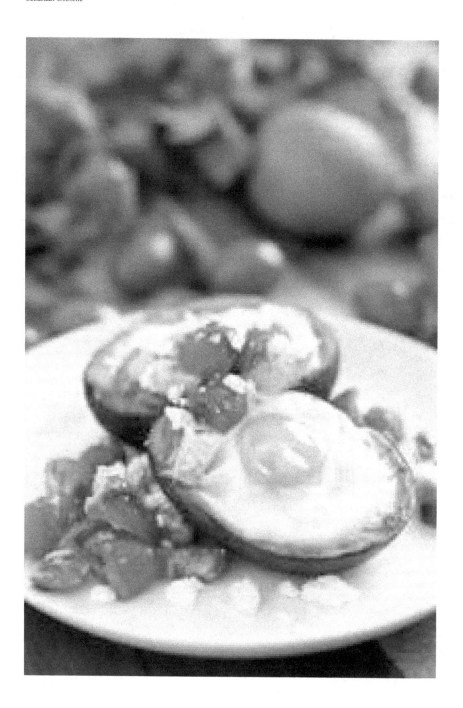

Sweet Potato Toast

Prep:

5 mins

Cook:

20 mins

Total:

25 mins

Servings:

4

Yield:

8 pieces

Ingredients

¼ cup mashed sweet potatoes

4 eggs

⅛ teaspoon ground nutmeg

8 slices whole wheat bread

⅛ teaspoon ground cinnamon

Directions

1

Whisk together the sweet potato, eggs, cinnamon, and nutmeg until smooth. Dip the bread into the egg mixture on both sides for several seconds until the bread is moist all the way through.

2

Heat a large, lightly-oiled skillet over medium heat. Cook the French toast in batches until golden brown on each side and no longer wet in the center, about 4 minutes per side.

Nutrition

Per Serving: 229 calories; protein 14g; carbohydrates 27.6g; fat 6.9g; cholesterol 186mg; sodium 350.1mg.

Greek Yogurt Oat Pancakes

Prep:

10 mins

Cook:

5 mins

Total:

15 mins

Servings:

4

Yield:

4 servings

Ingredients

6 ounces Greek yogurt

1 egg

½ cup all-purpose flour

1 teaspoon baking soda

Directions

1

Whisk yogurt in a bowl until smooth creamy; add egg and whisk to combine.

2

Whisk flour and baking soda together in a bowl; add to yogurt mixture and stir until smooth.

3

Heat a lightly oiled griddle over medium-high heat. Drop batter by large spoonfuls onto the griddle and cook until bubbles form and the edges are dry, 3 to 4 minutes. Flip and cook until browned on the other side, 2 to 3 minutes. Repeat with remaining batter.

Nutritions

Per Serving: 128 calories; protein 5.5g; carbohydrates 13.7g; fat 5.5g; cholesterol 50.5mg; sodium 358mg.

CHAPTER 2: LUNCH

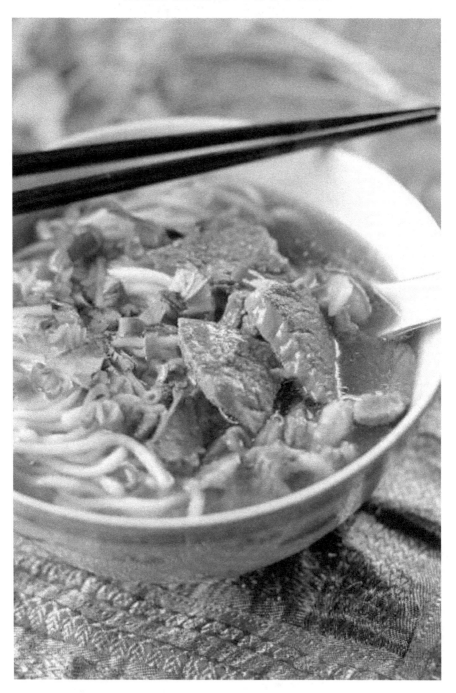

Beef Soup

Prep:

10 mins

Cook:

50 mins

Total:

1 hr

Servings:

8

Yield:

8 servings

Ingredients

1 pound ground beef

2 quarts water

1 (16 ounce) package frozen mixed vegetables

1 onion, chopped

4 potatoes, peeled and cubed

8 cubes beef bouillon, crumbled

½ teaspoon ground black pepper

1 (14.5 ounce) can diced tomatoes

Directions

1

In a large pot over medium heat, cook beef until brown; drain.

2

In a large pot over medium heat, combine cooked beef, water, tomatoes, onion, potatoes, mixed vegetables, bouillon and pepper. Bring to a boil, then reduce heat and simmer 45 minutes.

Nutrition

Per Serving: 254 calories; protein 14.6g; carbohydrates 30.5g; fat 8.3g; cholesterol 34.4mg; sodium 1014.1mg.

Apple Chicken

Prep:

10 mins

Cook:

20 mins

Total:

30 mins

Servings:

4

Yield:

4 servings

Ingredients

1 link Apple Chicken Sausage, sliced

1 quart fresh strawberries, hulled and quartered

1 medium Granny Smith apple, cored and cut into chunks

2 tablespoons honey

⅓ cup walnut pieces, toasted

¼ cup crumbled low-fat feta cheese

1 (5 ounce) package pre-washed spring mixed greens

2 tablespoons cider vinegar

1 tablespoon canola oil

Directions

1

In a non-stick skillet, over medium heat, lightly brown sausage. Set aside. In a large salad bowl, combine salad greens, strawberries, apple, walnuts, cheese and sausage.

2

In a small bowl, combine vinegar, honey and oil. Pour over salad and toss. Serve.

Nutrition

Per Serving: 272 calories; protein 7.9g; carbohydrates 29.5g; fat 15.6g; cholesterol 23.3mg; sodium 321.6mg.

Onion Tilapia

Prep:

10 mins

Cook:

15 mins

Additional:

2 mins

Total:

27 mins

Servings:

1

Yield:

1 tilapia fillet

Ingredients

¼ large lemon

1 (6 ounce) tilapia fillet, patted dry

1 tablespoon grated fresh Parmesan cheese

¼ large red onion, coarsely chopped

1 teaspoon minced garlic

1 teaspoon butter, divided

salt and ground black pepper to taste

1 tablespoon extra-virgin olive oil

Directions

1

Squeeze lemon juice over tilapia; season lightly with salt and black pepper.

2

Heat olive oil in a nonstick skillet over medium heat. Melt 1/2 teaspoon butter in hot oil. Add chopped onion and minced garlic; cook and stir until onion begins to look translucent, about 5 minutes.

3

Reduce heat to medium-low. Push onion mixture to sides of the skillet. Melt remaining 1/2 teaspoon of butter in the skillet. Place tilapia in the center of the skillet and cover with onion mixture. Cover skillet and cook tilapia until it starts to turn golden, about 5 minutes. Push onion mixture to the sides again and flip tilapia. Cover and cook until second side is golden and flakes easily with a fork, about 6 minutes more.

4

Remove skillet from heat. Top tilapia with grated Parmesan cheese, cover, and let stand until cheese is melted, about 3 minutes.

Nutrition

Per Serving: 371 calories; protein 37.3g; carbohydrates 7.6g; fat 21.4g; cholesterol 76.7mg; sodium 337.8mg.

Yogurt Soup

Prep:

10 mins

Cook:

25 mins

Total:

35 mins

Servings:

4

Yield:

4 servings

Ingredients

4 cups whole milk

3 cups plain yogurt

5 tablespoons all-purpose flour

2 cups water

2 egg yolks

4 teaspoons chicken bouillon granules

1 teaspoon salt

½ teaspoon ground black pepper

2 tablespoons lemon juice

Directions

1

Beat milk, yogurt, egg yolks, and all-purpose flour in a large bowl with an electric mixer.

2

Meanwhile, bring water and chicken bouillon to a boil in a large soup pot. Reduce heat to medium-low and add yogurt mixture, lemon juice, salt, and pepper, stirring occasionally until mixture thickens, about 20 minutes.

Nutrition

Per Serving: 332 calories; protein 20.2g; carbohydrates 32.9g; fat 13.4g; cholesterol 138.1mg; sodium 1187.2mg.

Tofu Parmigiana

Prep:

25 mins

Cook:

20 mins

Total:

45 mins

Servings:

4

Yield:

4 servings

Ingredients

½ cup seasoned bread crumbs

5 tablespoons grated Parmesan cheese

salt to taste

ground black pepper to taste

1 (12 ounce) package firm tofu

2 tablespoons olive oil

2 teaspoons dried oregano, divided

1 (8 ounce) can tomato sauce

1 clove garlic, minced

4 ounces shredded mozzarella cheese

½ teaspoon dried basil

Directions

1

In a small bowl, combine bread crumbs, 2 tablespoons Parmesan cheese, 1 teaspoon oregano, salt, and black pepper.

2

Slice tofu into 1/4 inch thick slices, and place in bowl of cold water. One at a time, press tofu slices into crumb mixture, turning to coat all sides.

3

Heat oil in a medium skillet over medium heat. Cook tofu slices until crisp on one side. Drizzle with a bit more olive oil, turn, and brown on the other side.

4

Combine tomato sauce, basil, garlic, and remaining oregano. Place a thin layer of sauce in an 8 inch square baking pan. Arrange tofu slices in the pan. Spoon remaining sauce over tofu. Top with shredded mozzarella and remaining 3 tablespoons Parmesan.

5

Bake at 400 degrees F for 20-22 minutes.

Nutrition

Per Serving: 357 calories; protein 25.7g; carbohydrates 18.8g; fat 21.5g; cholesterol 23.8mg; sodium 840.7mg.

Salmon Salad

Prep:

20 mins

Total:

20 mins

Servings:

6

Yield:

6 servings

Ingredients

2 cups mayonnaise

1 (3 ounce) package smoked salmon, flaked

½ lemon, juiced

2 tablespoons chopped capers

2 Granny Smith apples, cored and sliced

1 ½ cups sweet corn

3 tablespoons chopped fresh dill

Directions

1

Mix mayonnaise, lemon juice, dill, and capers together in a large bowl until smooth. Add apples, corn, and smoked salmon; toss gently until evenly coated. Chill before serving.

Nutrition

Per Serving: 603 calories; protein 4.9g; carbohydrates 17.8g; fat 59.2g; cholesterol 31.1mg; sodium 615.7mg.

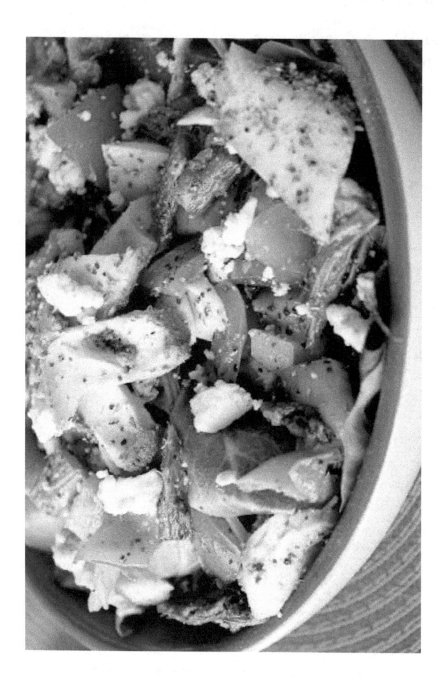

Pumpkin Coconut Milk Soup

Prep:

20 mins

Cook:

25 mins

Total:

45 mins

Servings:

5

Yield:

5 servings

Ingredients

2 tablespoons butter

1 onion, chopped

2 cups water

2 chicken bouillon cubes

2 (14 ounce) cans pumpkin puree

1 (14 ounce) can coconut milk

2 teaspoons ground ginger

1 teaspoon minced garlic

2 tablespoons orange juice

1 ½ teaspoons chili powder

1 ½ teaspoons pumpkin pie spice

Directions

1

Melt the butter in a large pot over medium heat; cook and stir the onion and garlic in the melted butter until softened, about 5 minutes.

Stir the water and chicken bouillon cubes into the mixture; cook and stir until the bouillon cubes have dissolved, 2 to 3 minutes. Stir the pumpkin puree, coconut milk, ginger, orange juice, pumpkin pie spice, and chili powder into the liquid. Bring the soup to a simmer, and cook until heated through, 5 to 7 minutes.

2

Pour the soup into a blender pitcher to no more than half full. Hold down the lid of the blender firmly in place. Start the blender, using a few quick pulses to get the soup moving before leaving it on to puree. Puree in batches until smooth, and pour into a clean pot. Alternately, you can use a stick blender and puree the soup in the pot.

3

Return the pureed soup to medium heat; bring to a simmer and cook another 10 minutes.

Nutrition

Per Serving: 282 calories; protein 4.4g; carbohydrates 21.9g; fat 22.2g; cholesterol 12.5mg; sodium 899.6mg.

Chicken Packets

Prep:

20 mins

Cook:

30 mins

Total:

50 mins

Servings:

4

Yield:

4 servings

Ingredients

4 skinless, boneless chicken breast halves

1 green bell pepper, seeded and sliced into strips

1 (20 ounce) can pineapple chunks, drained

1 red bell pepper, seeded and sliced into strips

1 onion, chopped

1 cup bottled teriyaki sauce or marinade

Directions

1

Preheat a grill for medium-high heat.

2

Lay out four squares of aluminum foil. Place one piece of chicken in the center of each square. Pour the teriyaki sauce over them, turning to coat. Distribute equal amounts of the green and red peppers, onion and pineapple chunks amongst the chicken pieces. Fold the foil up and seal tightly into packets.

3

Place the packets on the grill, and cook for about 20 minutes, or until chicken is no longer pink and juices run clear. I like to take one packet off the grill and check it before removing them all.

Nutrition

Per Serving: 304 calories; protein 33g; carbohydrates 38.9g; fat 1.7g; cholesterol 68.4mg; sodium 2841mg.

Iceberg Salad

Prep:

10 mins

Additional:

15 mins

Total:

25 mins

Servings:

4

Yield:

4 servings

Ingredients

3 large radishes, finely sliced

1 small head iceberg lettuce, chopped

¾ teaspoon salt

3 tablespoons rapeseed oil

1 tablespoon lemon juice

1 tablespoon unfiltered apple juice

¾ teaspoon white sugar

2 tablespoons cider vinegar

Directions

1

Combine radish and salt in a bowl and allow to sit for 15 minutes. Add oil, vinegar, lemon juice, apple juice, and sugar; mix well. Fold in iceberg lettuce until combined.

Nutrition

Per Serving: 111 calories; protein 0.8g; carbohydrates 4.5g; fat 10.3g; sodium 449.9mg.

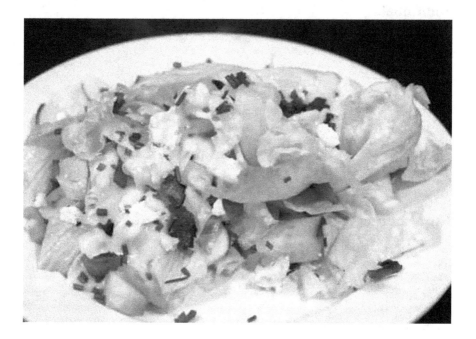

Spiced Rub

Prep:

5 mins

Total:

5 mins

Servings:

8

Yield:

1 1/4 cup

Ingredients

½ cup brown sugar

1 tablespoon garlic powder

½ cup paprika

1 tablespoon salt

1 tablespoon chili powder

1 tablespoon onion powder

1 tablespoon ground black pepper

Directions

1

Mix brown sugar, paprika, black pepper, salt, chili powder, garlic powder, onion powder, and cayenne pepper in a bowl. Store in an airtight container or keep in the freezer in a sealable plastic bag.

Nutrition

Per Serving: 66 calories; protein 1.5g; carbohydrates 15.3g; fat 1.1g; sodium 888.1mg.

Broccoli Ziti

Prep:

30 mins

Cook:

1 hr

Total:

1 hr 30 mins

Servings:

8

Yield:

8 servings

Ingredients

1 pound dry ziti pasta

salt and pepper to taste

3 cloves garlic, chopped

¼ cup grated Parmesan cheese

2 tablespoons butter

1 pint heavy cream

1 cube chicken bouillon

3 tablespoons cornstarch

2 large heads broccoli, steamed

1 (14 ounce) can artichoke hearts in water

6 breaded and fried skinless, boneless chicken breast halves, chopped

1 (10.75 ounce) can chicken broth

Directions

1

In a large pot of salted boiling water, place pasta and cook for 8 to 10 minutes, until pasta is al dente. Drain.

2

In a large skillet, saute garlic in butter over medium heat. Stir in the heavy cream, chicken broth, and bouillon. Add Parmesan cheese, salt, and pepper. Add cornstarch (adjust amount to thicken sauce to your liking). Simmer all together for about 20 minutes.

3

Once sauce is cooked and thickens, add broccoli and artichoke hearts, stir all together and cook for another 2 to 3 minutes. Once sauce is done, put cooked ziti pasta in a large bowl, pour sauce over pasta and toss to coat and mix. Then add the chicken pieces and mix all together.

Nutrition

Per Serving: 820 calories; protein 42.3g; carbohydrates 69.3g; fat 41.6g; cholesterol 180.7mg; sodium 1076.9mg.

Pork Tenderloin with Mustard Sauce

Prep:

15 mins

Cook:

1 hr

Additional:

8 hrs

Total:

9 hrs 15 mins

Servings:

8

Yield:

8 servings

Ingredients

1 ½ tablespoons mustard powder

⅓ cup red wine

2 tablespoons light brown sugar

⅓ cup soy sauce

2 pounds pork tenderloin

⅓ cup mayonnaise

⅓ cup sour cream

Directions

1

Combine wine, soy sauce, and brown sugar in a large resealable plastic bag. Place tenderloin in bag, and refrigerate overnight, or at least 8 hours.

2

In a small bowl, combine mayonnaise, sour cream, mustard powder; mix well. Mix in minced chives if you wish. Chill until ready to serve.

3

Preheat oven to 325 degrees F. Place meat and marinade in a shallow baking dish, and roast for 1 hour, basting occasionally. Temperature of meat should register 145 degrees F. Let rest for a few minutes, then cut into 1/2 inch thick slices. Serve with mustard sauce.

Nutrition

Per Serving: 259 calories; protein 25g; carbohydrates 5.5g; fat 13.9g; cholesterol 81.4mg; sodium 718.8mg.

Cod Curry

Prep:

15 mins

Cook:

55 mins

Total:

1 hr 10 mins

Servings:

4

Yield:

4 servings

Ingredients

2 tablespoons vegetable oil

1 medium onion, chopped

1 teaspoon garlic paste

1 teaspoon ginger paste

2 teaspoons cumin

2 teaspoons coriander

1 teaspoon cardamom

½ teaspoon turmeric

½ teaspoon salt

2 fresh jalapeno peppers, seeded and diced

.24 cup chopped cilantro

1 tablespoon lemon juice

1 (28 ounce) can diced tomatoes with juice

1 pound cod fillets, cut into chunks

Directions

1

Heat the oil in a skillet over medium heat. Place onion in the skillet. Reduce heat to low, and cook, stirring often, 15 minutes, or until soft and brown.

2

Mix the garlic paste and ginger paste into the skillet. Cook 1 minute. Mix in cumin, coriander, cardamom, turmeric, and salt. Stir in the jalapeno, cilantro, lemon juice, and tomatoes with juice, scraping up any brown bits from the bottom of the skillet. Bring to a boil. Reduce heat to low, cover, and simmer 20 minutes. If you like, the sauce may be set aside for a few hours at this point to allow the flavors to blend.

3

Return the sauce to a boil, and place cod in the skillet. Reduce heat to low, and cook 15 minutes, or until fish flakes easily with a fork.

Nutritions

Per Serving: 227 calories; protein 23.6g; carbohydrates 11.4g; fat 8.4g; cholesterol 52.8mg; sodium 757mg.

Fish Stew

Prep:

45 mins

Cook:

45 mins

Total:

1 hr 30 mins

Servings:

6

Yield:

6 servings

Ingredients

¼ cup olive oil

2 leeks, coarsely chopped

1 large onion, chopped

1 bulb fennel bulb, coarsely chopped

5 cloves garlic, minced

1 quart fish stock

2 cups vermouth

1 cup canned diced tomatoes

1 red bell pepper - stemmed, seeded, and diced

1 orange, zested

¼ teaspoon red pepper flakes

freshly ground pepper to taste

1 bay leaf

1 ½ pounds boneless cod fillets, cut into bite-size pieces

½ pound shrimp, peeled and deveined

½ pound clams, scrubbed

½ pound mussels, scrubbed

Directions

1

Heat olive oil in a large pot over medium heat. Add leeks and onion; cook and stir until softened, 8 to 10 minutes. Add fennel and garlic; cook and stir until fragrant, about 5 minutes.

2

Pour fish stock and vermouth into the pot. Add tomatoes, red bell pepper, orange zest, red pepper flakes, pepper, and bay leaf. Bring to a boil; reduce heat, cover, and simmer until red bell pepper is soft, about 20 minutes.

3

Bring stock back to a boil. Add cod fillets; cook for 1 minute. Add shrimp, clams, and mussels; cook, shaking pot occasionally, until shells open and shrimp turn opaque, 1 to 2 minutes.

Nutritions

Per Serving: 511 calories; protein 47g; carbohydrates 28.5g; fat 13.5g; cholesterol 146.5mg; sodium 875mg.

CHAPTER 3: DINNER

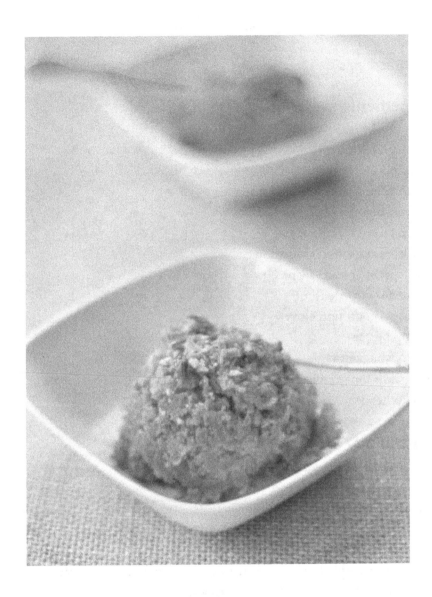

Carrot Pudding

Servings:

7

Yield:

6 to 8 servings

Ingredients

1 cup grated carrots
1 teaspoon baking soda
1 cup peeled and shredded potatoes
1 cup white sugar
1 cup raisins
1 teaspoon ground cinnamon
1 teaspoon ground allspice
1 cup all-purpose flour
1 teaspoon ground cloves
½ cup butter
1 cup white sugar
1 ½ teaspoons vanilla extract
½ cup heavy whipping cream

Directions

1

In a large mixing bowl, combine carrots, potatoes, sugar, raisins, flour, baking soda, ground cinnamon, all spice, and ground cloves. Transfer mixture to a clean 1 pound coffee can. Secure wax paper over the top and place the filled can in a large pot with 2 to 3 inches of water. Cover the pot and bring the water to a simmer.

2

Steam the cake for 2 hours. Serve warm.

3

Buttery sauce: In a medium-size pot, combine butter or margarine, cream, sugar, and vanilla. Heat until the mixture is liquid. Spoon mixture over the warm carrot pudding to serve.

Nutrition

Per Serving: 552 calories; protein 3.6g; carbohydrates 93.8g; fat 19.9g; cholesterol 58.2mg; sodium 295.5mg.

Paprika Tilapia

Prep:

10 mins

Cook:

8 mins

Total:

18 mins

Servings:

4

Yield:

4 servings

Ingredients

3 tablespoons olive oil

½ teaspoon freshly ground black pepper

1 teaspoon garlic powder

½ teaspoon salt

4 (6 ounce) tilapia fillets

cooking spray

2 teaspoons ground smoked paprika

Directions

1

Combine olive oil, paprika, garlic powder, salt, and black pepper in a small bowl; stir well. Brush oil mixture evenly over tilapia fillets.

2

Heat a large nonstick grill pan over medium-high heat; grease with cooking spray. Grill fish until it flakes easily with a fork, about 4 minutes per side.

Nutrition

Per Serving: 264 calories; protein 34.8g; carbohydrates 1.3g; fat 12.5g; cholesterol 61.6mg; sodium 367.2mg.

Fried Rice

Prep:

10 mins

Cook:

30 mins

Additional:

20 mins

Total:

1 hr

Servings:

6

Yield:

6 servings

Ingredients

1 ½ cups uncooked jasmine rice

3 tablespoons oyster sauce

3 cups water

2 teaspoons canola oil

1 (12 ounce) can fully cooked luncheon meat (such as SPAM®), cubed

½ cup sliced Chinese sweet pork sausage (lup cheong)

3 eggs, beaten

1 (8 ounce) can pineapple chunks, drained

½ cup chopped green onion

2 tablespoons canola oil

½ teaspoon garlic powder

Directions

1

Bring the rice and water to a boil in a saucepan over high heat. Reduce heat to medium-low, cover, and simmer until the rice is tender, and the liquid has been absorbed, 20 to 25 minutes. Let the rice cool completely.

2

Heat 2 teaspoons of oil in a skillet over medium heat, and brown the luncheon meat and sausage. Set aside, and pour the beaten eggs into the hot skillet. Scramble the eggs, and set aside.

3

Heat 2 tablespoons of oil in a large nonstick skillet over medium heat, and stir in the rice. Toss the rice with the hot oil until heated through and beginning to brown, about 2 minutes. Add the garlic powder, toss the rice for 1 more minute to develop the garlic taste, and stir in the luncheon meat, sausage, scrambled eggs, pineapple, and oyster sauce. Cook and stir until the oyster sauce coats the rice and other

Ingredients, 2 to 3 minutes, stir in the green onions, and serve.

Nutrition

Per Serving: 511 calories; protein 17.1g; carbohydrates 48g; fat 28.1g; cholesterol 132.7mg; sodium 988.1mg.

Pasta with Pumpkin Sauce

Prep:

10 mins

Cook:

30 mins

Total:

40 mins

Servings:

4

Yield:

4 servings

Ingredients

¼ cup butter, divided

salt and freshly ground black pepper to taste

1 pound sugar pumpkin - peeled, seeded, and cut into small cubes

½ pound orecchiette pasta

1 cup heavy cream

4 tablespoons Parmesan cheese

2 orange bell peppers, seeded and diced

1 onion, minced

Directions

1

Melt 1/2 the butter in a large skillet over medium-low heat and cook onion until soft and translucent, about 5 minutes. Add pumpkin and cook for 2 minutes. Cover, reduce heat, and cook, stirring often, until soft, about 28-30 minutes.

2

Meanwhile, bring a large pot of lightly salted water to a boil. Cook orecchiette in the boiling water, stirring occasionally until almost tender yet firm to the bite, about 10 minutes, 2 minutes less than indicated on the package. Drain and transfer to a bowl.

3

Melt the remaining butter in a second skillet and cook bell peppers until softened, 5 to 10 minutes. Add to the bowl with the cooked pasta.

4

Once pumpkin is tender, add cream and Parmesan cheese to skillet. Season with salt and pepper and stir until smooth. Add drained pasta and cooked bell peppers and mix well.

Nutrition

Per Serving: 581 calories; protein 12g; carbohydrates 55.5g; fat 36.1g; cholesterol 116.4mg; sodium 222.9mg.

Herbed Sole

Prep:

15 mins

Cook:

30 mins

Total:

45 mins

Servings:

4

Yield:

4 servings

Ingredients

1 tablespoon lemon juice

1 tablespoon all-purpose flour

2 tablespoons thinly sliced green onion

1 clove garlic, minced

¼ cup dry white wine

4 (6 ounce) fillets sole

salt to taste

ground black pepper to taste

¼ teaspoon paprika

¼ pound cooked salad shrimp

2 tablespoons butter

Directions

1

In a small bowl, combine lemon juice, green onion, garlic, and wine. Set aside.

2

Lay filets flat, and divide shrimp evenly among them in a band across one end of each fillet. Roll up around shrimp, and secure with toothpick. Place in a baking dish. Season to taste with salt, pepper, and paprika. Pour lemon juice mixture over the fish. Cover.

3

Bake at 350 degrees F for 25 minutes.

4

When fillets are nearly done, prepare sauce. In a small saucepan, melt butter over medium heat. Stir in flour. Transfer fish to serving platter ,and keep warm. Pour pan juices into butter/flour mixture; cook and stir until thickened. Pour over sole, and serve.

Nutrition

Per Serving: 253 calories; protein 37.5g; carbohydrates 2.8g; fat 8.1g; cholesterol 149.9mg; sodium 226.5mg.

Egg Cheese Quiche

Prep:

30 mins

Cook:

1 hr

Total:

1 hr 30 mins

Servings:

6

Yield:

1 (9 inch) quiche

Ingredients

1 tablespoon butter

1 (12 ounce) package spicy ground pork sausage

4 eggs

1 (8 ounce) package Cheddar cheese, shredded

½ cup Ranch-style salad dressing

½ cup milk

1 dash hot pepper sauce

salt and pepper to taste

1 pinch white sugar

1 (9 inch) unbaked deep dish pie crust

½ onion, chopped

Directions

1

Preheat oven to 425 degrees F.

2

Heat butter in a large skillet over medium heat. Saute onion until soft. Add sausage, and cook until evenly brown. Drain, crumble, and set aside.

3

In a medium bowl, whisk together eggs, Ranch dressing and milk. Stir in shredded cheese. Season with hot sauce, salt, pepper and sugar.

4

Spread sausage mixture in the bottom of crust. Cover with egg mixture, and shake lightly to remove air, and to level contents.

5

Bake in preheated oven for 15 to 20 minutes. Reduce heat to 350 degrees F, and bake 45 to 50 minutes, or until filling is puffed and golden brown. Remove from oven, prick top with a knife, and let cool 10 minutes before serving.

Nutrition

Per Serving: 718 calories; protein 22.5g; carbohydrates 19.3g; fat 60.9g; cholesterol 213.4mg; sodium 1450.6mg.

Squash Soup

Servings:

8

Yield:

8 servings

Ingredients

2 tablespoons olive oil

1 tablespoon plain yogurt

1 (3 pound) butternut squash - peeled, seeded, and cubed

4 cups vegetable broth

2 sweet potatoes, peeled and cubed

3 apples, peeled and cubed

1 large onion, coarsely chopped

3 large cloves garlic, crushed

½ teaspoon ground cinnamon

¼ teaspoon ground nutmeg

¼ teaspoon ground cumin

¼ teaspoon ground ginger

1 teaspoon salt

¼ teaspoon ground black pepper

1 pint half-and-half

Directions

1

Heat olive oil in a pressure cooker over medium-high heat. Saute onion until translucent but not browned, about 5 minutes. Add squash, broth, sweet potatoes, apples, garlic, cinnamon, nutmeg, black pepper, cumin, ginger, and salt.

2

Close and lock the lid. Bring to high pressure according to manufacturer's instructions, 10 to 15 minutes. Reduce heat to medium-low; cook until squash and sweet potatoes are fork-tender, about 15 minutes.

3

Release pressure carefully using the quick-release method according to manufacturer's instructions. Unlock and remove lid. Liquefy soup using an immersion blender. Stir in half-and-half. Serve with a dollop of yogurt on top.

Nutrition

Per Serving: 313 calories; protein 6g; carbohydrates 49.6g; fat 12.1g; cholesterol 26mg; sodium 598.4mg.

Cumin Chicken

Prep:

30 mins

Cook:

53 mins

Total:

1 hr 23 mins

Servings:

8

Yield:

8 servings

Ingredients

2 ½ cups coarsely chopped onions

¼ cup coarsely chopped garlic

¼ cup chopped peeled ginger

2 cups long-grain white rice

2 ½ teaspoons salt

20 chicken wings, tips removed and sections separated

1 ½ tablespoons ground cumin

2 tablespoons olive oil

2 cups chopped cilantro stems, divided

1 (14 ounce) can diced tomatoes

1 tablespoon sriracha sauce

2 ½ cups water

Directions

1

Heat olive oil in a pot large enough to hold chicken wings in a single layer. Add chicken wings; cook until browned, about 8 minutes. Turn wings with tongs; cook until second side is browned, about 8 minutes more. Transfer to a bowl using tongs.

2

Stir onions, garlic, and ginger into the drippings in the pot; cook until fragrant, 2 to 3 minutes. Stir in rice and cumin. Add water, 1 1/2 cup cilantro stems, tomatoes, sriracha sauce, and salt.

3

Return wings to the pot. Bring broth to a boil. Cover, reduce heat to low, and simmer until rice and wings are tender, about 30 minutes. Garnish with remaining 1/2 cup cilantro stems.

Nutrition

Per Serving: 388 calories; protein 18.1g; carbohydrates 46.3g; fat 13.8g; cholesterol 40.3mg; sodium 937.4mg.

Chili Tuna

Prep:

20 mins

Total:

20 mins

Servings:

6

Yield:

6 servings

Ingredients

2 (5 ounce) cans tuna, drained

1 tablespoon water

⅔ tablespoon sweet chili sauce

1 (8 ounce) package Neufchatel cheese

6 green onions, chopped

6 (12 inch) flour tortillas

Directions

1

In a small bowl, mix tuna, chili sauce and green onions. Blend in enough water to allow easy spreading.

2

Lay tortillas one by one on a flat surface. Spread a thin layer of cheese onto each tortilla, covering the entire surface. Spread tuna mixture over cheese to within an inch of tortilla edge.

3

Starting at the top, roll up the tortilla into a snug cylindrical shape, ensuring the cream cheese seals the bottom.

4

Enclose roll-ups in aluminum foil, and refrigerate or freeze until serving. When ready to serve, cut the roll-ups into 2 inch slices. If frozen, slice the roll-ups about 13-15 minutes before serving time to allow them to defrost completely.

Nutrition

Per Serving: 518 calories; protein 24.4g; carbohydrates 63g; fat 18.2g; cholesterol 41mg; sodium 935.4mg.

Fettuccine with Asparagus

Prep:

10 mins

Cook:

20 mins

Total:

30 mins

Servings:

3

Yield:

3 servings

Ingredients

½ bunch asparagus, trimmed and cut into 1/2-inch pieces

1 cup frozen peas

1 (1 ounce) slice prosciutto, cut into thin strips

¼ cup water

3 tablespoons butter

2 cups whole milk

2 teaspoons garlic powder

1 cup freshly grated Parmesan cheese

1 pinch salt and ground black pepper to taste

3 tablespoons all-purpose flour

4 ounces dry fettuccine pasta

Directions

1

Combine the asparagus, peas, and water in a saucepan over medium heat. Cover the saucepan and cook until the vegetables are beginning to become tender, yet retain some crispness, about 5 minutes; drain any remaining liquid and set the vegetables aside.

2

Melt the butter in the saucepan over medium-low heat. Stir the flour into the butter until combined, 2 to 4 minutes. Add the milk, raise heat to medium and cook, whisking frequently, until the mixture thickens, another 2 to 3 minutes. Stir the garlic powder and Parmesan cheese into the sauce; season with salt and pepper. Set aside.

3

Bring a pot of lightly salted water to a boil. Cook the fettuccine in the boiling water until the pasta is cooked yet firm to the bite, about 8 minutes; drain and return the fettuccine to the pot. Stir the vegetables, the sauce, and the prosciutto into the fettuccine.

Nutrition

Per Serving: 556 calories; protein 28g; carbohydrates 53g; fat 26.6g; cholesterol 75.4mg; sodium 854.2mg.

Fresh Calamari

Prep:

15 mins

Cook:

10 mins

Total:

25 mins

Servings:

8

Yield:

8 servings

Ingredients

½ cup olive oil

2 cloves garlic, pressed

¼ cup red wine vinegar

1 cup water

1 pound squid, cleaned and cut into rings and tentacles

1 cup chopped celery

½ bunch chopped fresh cilantro

1 green bell pepper, chopped

1 red bell pepper, chopped

1 cup dry white wine

1 yellow bell pepper, chopped

1 cup chopped cucumber

1 bunch chopped fresh parsley

1 cup jicama, peeled and shredded

1 bunch fresh green onions, chopped

1 jalapeno pepper, finely chopped

Directions

1

In a small bowl, mix the olive oil, red wine vinegar, and garlic.

2

In a medium saucepan, bring the wine and water to a low boil. Stir in the squid and cook until opaque, about 2-3 minutes. Drain and cool.

3

In a large bowl, mix the celery, cilantro, green bell pepper, red bell pepper, yellow bell pepper, cucumber, green onions, parsley, jicama, and jalapeno. Toss gently with the squid and the olive oil dressing mixture. Chill until serving.

Nutrition

Per Serving: 236 calories; protein 10.5g; carbohydrates 10.9g; fat 14.6g; cholesterol 132.2mg; sodium 51.6mg.

Nicoise Salad

Prep:

20 mins

Total:

20 mins

Servings:

4

Yield:

4 servings

Ingredients

Dressing:

2 tablespoons Dijon mustard

1 teaspoon sugar

1 tablespoon chopped fresh parsley

½ cup extra-virgin olive oil

⅓ cup red wine vinegar

Salt and ground black pepper to taste

Salad:

1 (14.5 ounce) can whole potatoes, drained and halved

1 (14 ounce) can artichoke hearts, well drained and quartered

1 (14 ounce) can sliced hearts of palm, drained

1 (14.5 ounce) can French-style no salt added green beans, drained

1 (5 ounce) can tuna packed in water, drained and gently flaked

1 large tomato, cut into wedges

2 hard-cooked eggs, cut into wedges

1 (2.2 ounce) can sliced black olives, drained

Directions

1

Prepare Dressing: In small bowl combine mustard, red wine vinegar, parsley and sugar: gradually whisk in olive oil until well blended. Add salt and pepper to taste.

2

Prepare Salad: On large platter arrange potatoes, green beans, artichoke hearts, hearts of palm, tuna, olives, tomato wedges and hard-cooked eggs. Drizzle salad with dressing.

Nutrition

Per Serving: 490 calories; protein 18.5g; carbohydrates 30.7g; fat 33.4g; cholesterol 115.4mg; sodium 1757.9mg.

Pork Chili

Prep:

15 mins

Cook:

3 hrs 50 mins

Total:

4 hrs 5 mins

Servings:

10

Yield:

10 servings

Ingredients

cooking spray

1 sweet onion (such as Vidalia®), chopped

1 (15.5 ounce) can canned chili starter (such as BUSH'S Chili Magic®)

2 tablespoons dried oregano

2 cups chicken broth

½ sweet onion (such as Vidalia®), chopped

1 green bell pepper, chopped

1 jalapeno pepper, minced

2 teaspoons ground cumin

1 ½ tablespoons unsweetened cocoa powder

1 ½ tablespoons chili powder

2 teaspoons garlic salt

2 teaspoons paprika

1 teaspoon cayenne pepper

1 ¼ pounds ground lean turkey

1 pound lean ground pork

1 (28 ounce) can diced tomatoes with green chile peppers (such as RO*TEL®)
1 (14.5 ounce) can fire-roasted diced tomatoes with garlic
1 (14.5 ounce) can diced tomatoes with green peppers and onions

Directions

1

Coat a large saucepan with cooking spray and cook 1 chopped sweet onion over medium heat until tender, about 5 minutes. Add chili starter, oregano, and chicken broth; increase heat to medium-high and simmer for 20 minutes.

2

Coat a large stock pot with cooking spay and cook remaining 1/2 chopped sweet onion, green bell pepper, and jalapeno pepper over medium heat until tender, 5 to 8 minutes. Add ground cumin, cocoa powder, chili powder, garlic salt, paprika, and cayenne pepper; cook 2 minutes. Mix in ground turkey and pork; cook and stir until meat is crumbly, evenly browned, and no longer pink, about 10 more minutes. Drain and discard any excess grease.

3

Stir diced tomatoes with green chiles, fire-roasted tomatoes, and diced tomatoes with green peppers and onions into chili; simmer for about 3 hours.

Nutritions

Per Serving: 272 calories; protein 23.3g; carbohydrates 18.1g; fat 11.9g; cholesterol 72.3mg; sodium 1409.4mg.

Flank Steak

Prep:

10 mins

Cook:

15 mins

Additional:

2 hrs 40 mins

Total:

3 hrs 5 mins

Servings:

8

Yield:

8 servings

Ingredients

1 medium orange, cut into quarters

1 lemon, juiced and zested

1 cup orange juice

¼ cup rice vinegar

¼ cup soy sauce

¼ cup maple syrup

¼ cup honey

4 cloves garlic

1 tablespoon grated fresh ginger root

1 tablespoon ground black pepper

1 teaspoon cayenne pepper

4 green onions, cut into 1/4-inch pieces

2 pounds flank steak

Directions

1

Combine orange pieces, lemon juice, lemon zest, orange juice, rice vinegar, soy sauce, maple syrup, honey, garlic cloves, ginger, pepper, and cayenne pepper in a blender; blend until marinade is smooth. Mix in green onions.

2

Place flank steak into a shallow baking dish and pour marinade over meat, making sure marinade gets underneath the meat as well. Cover the dish, refrigerate, and marinate for at least 2 hours, or overnight.

3

Remove steak from the refrigerator and allow to come to room temperature for at least 30 minutes before grilling. Lift up steak from the dish to let juices run off; reserve marinade.

4

Preheat an outdoor grill for medium-high heat and lightly oil the grate.

5

Cook flank steak on the preheated grill until it begins to firm and is reddish-pink and juicy in the center, 5 to 7 minutes per side. An instant-read thermometer inserted into the center should read 130 degrees F (54 degrees C).

6

Cover steak and set aside to rest for 10 minutes before slicing thinly against the grain.

7

While steak is resting, pour remaining marinade in a saucepan over medium-high heat and bring to a boil. Cook until sauce is reduced, about 5 minutes. Serve with the flank steak.

Nutritions

Per Serving: 197 calories; protein 15.1g; carbohydrates 24.9g; fat 4.9g; cholesterol 25.3mg; sodium 481.3mg.

CHAPTER 4: SNACK & APPETIZER

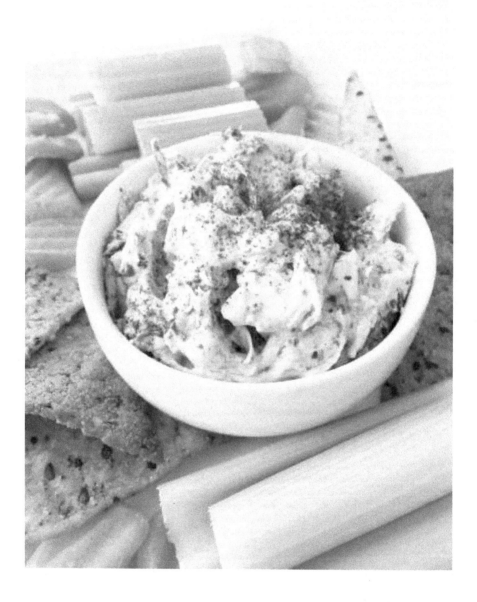

Artichoke Dip

Prep:

5 mins

Cook:

20 mins

Total:

25 mins

Servings:

7

Yield:

5 to 8 servings

Ingredients

½ cup mayonnaise

½ cup sour cream

salt and pepper to taste

1 (14 ounce) can artichoke hearts, drained

½ cup minced red onion

1 cup grated Parmesan cheese

1 tablespoon lemon juice

Directions

1

Preheat oven to 400 degrees F.

2

In a medium-sized mixing bowl, stir together mayonnaise, sour cream, Parmesan cheese and onion. When these ingredients are combined, mix in artichoke hearts, lemon juice, salt and pepper. Transfer mixture to a shallow baking dish.

3

Bake at 400 degrees F for 20 minutes, or until light brown on top.

Nutrition

Per Serving: 221 calories; protein 6.4g; carbohydrates 6.6g; fat 19.2g; cholesterol 23.3mg; sodium 481.4mg.

Walnuts Pesto

Prep:

10 mins

Total:

10 mins

Servings:

2

Yield:

2 servings

Ingredients

½ cup walnuts

2 cloves garlic

1 tablespoon lemon juice

¼ cup olive oil

2 cups basil leaves

Directions

1

Blend basil, walnuts, olive oil, garlic, and lemon juice together in a food processor until pesto has a paste-like consistency.

Nutrition

Per Serving: 455 calories; protein 6.1g; carbohydrates 6.9g; fat 47.3g; sodium 2.9mg.

Pearl Onions Snack

Prep:

5 mins

Cook:

25 mins

Total:

30 mins

Servings:

8

Yield:

8 servings

Ingredients

1 pound pearl onions
2 tablespoons chopped fresh parsley
3 tablespoons butter
1 pinch ground nutmeg
1 ½ cups light cream
½ teaspoon salt
ground black pepper to taste
3 tablespoons all-purpose flour

Directions

1

Place onions into a large pot and cover with salted water; bring to a boil. Reduce heat to medium-low and simmer until tender, about 10 minutes. Drain.

2

Melt butter in a large skillet over medium heat; cook and stir flour and nutmeg in melted butter for about 5 minutes; season with salt and pepper. Add cream to flour mixture; cook and stir until bubbly and thick, about 5 minutes more. Stir onion and parsley into cream sauce until heated through, 2 to 4 minutes.

Nutrition

Per Serving: 171 calories; protein 2.3g; carbohydrates 12.1g; fat 13.1g; cholesterol 41.1mg; sodium 204.7mg.

Mango Salsa

Prep:

15 mins

Additional:

30 mins

Total:

45 mins

Servings:

8

Yield:

8 servings

Ingredients

1 mango - peeled, seeded, and chopped
1 fresh jalapeno chile pepper, finely chopped
¼ cup finely chopped red bell pepper
1 green onion, chopped
2 tablespoons lime juice
1 tablespoon lemon juice
2 tablespoons chopped cilantro

Directions

1

In a medium bowl, mix mango, red bell pepper, green onion, cilantro, jalapeno, lime juice, and lemon juice. Cover, and allow to sit at least 30 minutes before serving.

Nutrition

Per Serving: 21 calories; protein 0.3g; carbohydrates 5.4g; fat 0.1g; sodium 1.4mg.

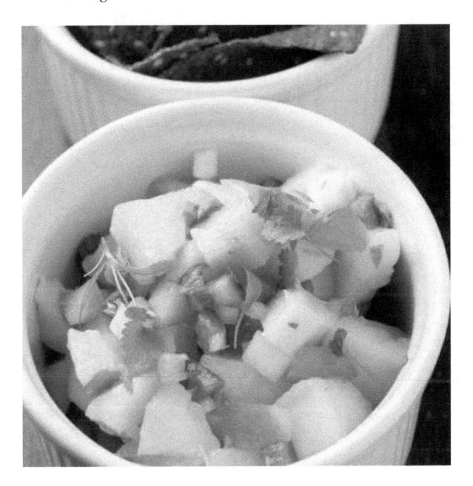

Bruschetta

Prep:

5 mins

Cook:

7 mins

Total:

12 mins

Servings:

6

Yield:

6 servings

Ingredients

1 French baguette

1 tablespoon olive oil

2 roma (plum) tomatoes, thinly sliced

1 tablespoon chopped fresh basil

1 tablespoon chopped fresh oregano

1 teaspoon garlic powder

1 pinch ground white pepper

1 (8 ounce) package sliced mozzarella cheese

1 (6 ounce) package sliced provolone cheese

Directions

1

Preheat oven to 350 degrees F (175 degrees C).

2

Slice the baguette into 1/2 inch thick diagonal slices. Arrange the slices in a single layer on a baking sheet. Brush both sides of each slice with the olive oil. Place tomato slices and a sprinkling of basil and oregano on the bread slices. Sprinkle the tomatoes, basil and oregano with the garlic powder and white pepper. Cover the tomato slices with slices of the mozzarella and provolone. Place more basil, oregano and tomato slices on top of the cheese.

3

Bake in the preheated oven for 7 to 10 minutes, or until the cheese is bubbly.

Nutritions

Per Serving: 439 calories; protein 25.5g; carbohydrates 45.7g; fat 17.2g; cholesterol 43.4mg; sodium 972.4mg.

CHAPTER 5: **SMOOTHIES & DRINKS**

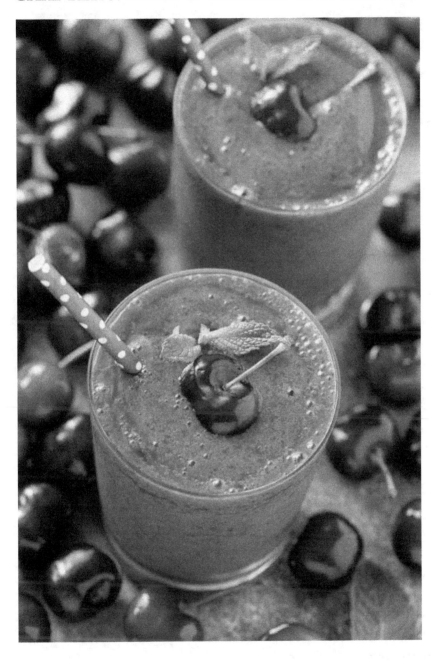

Berries Smoothie

Prep:

5 mins

Total:

5 mins

Servings:

2

Yield:

2 servings

Ingredients

1 cup Almond Breeze Vanilla or Unsweetened Vanilla almondmilk

½ cup fresh raspberries

½ cup fresh blueberries

½ cup fresh blackberries

Directions

1

Puree all Ingredients in a blender until smooth.

Nutrition:

Calories 100

Total Fat 1.5

Cholesterol 0mg

Sodium 75

Potassium 223mg

Total Carbohydrate 20g

Dietary Fiber 5g

Sugars 14g

Protein 2g

Vanille Kipferl

Prep:

30 mins

Cook:

8 mins

Additional:

2 mins

Total:

40 mins

Servings:

18

Yield:

3 dozen

Ingredients

2 cups all-purpose flour

¼ cup confectioners' sugar

⅓ cup white sugar

1 cup unsalted butter

¼ cup vanilla sugar

¾ cup ground almonds

Directions

1

Preheat oven to 325 degrees F. Line a baking sheet with parchment paper.

2

Combine flour, 1/3 cup sugar, and ground almonds. Cut in butter with pastry blender, then quickly knead into a dough.

3

Shape dough into logs and cut off 1/2-inch pieces. Shape each piece into a crescent and place on prepared baking sheet.

4

Bake in preheated oven until edges are golden brown, 8 to 10 minutes. Cool 1 minute and carefully roll in vanilla sugar mixture.

Nutrition

Per Serving: 207 calories; protein 2.8g; carbohydrates 20g; fat 13.4g; cholesterol 27.1mg; sodium 1.8mg.

Mango & Lime Smoothie

Prep:

10 mins

Total:

10 mins

Servings:

4

Yield:

4 servings

Ingredients

2 tablespoons confectioners' sugar

1 tray ice cubes

2 tablespoons fresh lime juice

3 mangoes, peeled, pitted, and cut into 1-inch chunks

Directions

1

Place the mangoes, lime juice, confectioners' sugar, and ice cubes in a blender. Blend until slushy.

Nutrition

Per Serving: 117 calories; protein 0.8g; carbohydrates 30.7g; fat 0.4g; sodium 5.8mg.

Mango Smoothie

Prep:

10 mins

Total:

10 mins

Servings:

1

Yield:

1 smoothie

Ingredients

½ mango, chopped

½ cup almond milk

½ cup ice

1 scoop vanilla whey protein powder

½ cup low-fat vanilla yogurt

Directions

1

Blend mango, yogurt, almond milk, ice, protein powder, and honey together in a blender until smooth.

Nutrition

Per Serving: 401 calories; protein 44.6g; carbohydrates 48.7g; fat 4.4g; cholesterol 18.6mg; sodium 379.4mg.

Avocado & Spinach Smoothie

Prep:

5 mins

Total:

5 mins

Servings:

2

Yield:

2 servings

Ingredients

½ cup coconut milk

½ cup water

ice cubes

½ cup fresh spinach

½ medium avocado, pitted and scooped from shell

2 tablespoons erythritol

½ teaspoon vanilla powder

1 tablespoon medium-chain triglyceride (MCT) oil

Directions

1

Combine coconut milk, water, ice cubes, avocado, spinach, erythritol, MCT oil, and vanilla powder in a blender. Blend until smooth.

Nutrition

Per Serving: 256 calories; protein 2.4g; carbohydrates 17.6g; fat 26.4g; sodium 19.5mg.

Banana Oat Smoothie

Prep:

10 mins

Total:

10 mins

Servings:

1

Yield:

1 serving

Ingredients

1 banana, broken in half

1 cup ice

¼ cup old-fashioned rolled oats

½ cup vanilla yogurt

½ cup skim milk

1 ½ tablespoons peanut butter

1 teaspoon honey, or to taste

1 teaspoon ground cinnamon, or to taste

Directions

1

Put banana, ice, oats, yogurt, skim milk, peanut butter, honey, and cinnamon, respectively, in a blender; blend until smooth.

Nutritions

Per Serving: 499 calories; protein 20.4g; carbohydrates 76.4g; fat 15.7g; cholesterol 8.6mg; sodium 254.6mg.

Beet Velvet Smoothie

Prep:

10 mins

Total:

10 mins

Servings:

1

Yield:

1 serving

Ingredients

1 cup fresh spinach

1 beet, peeled and cut into quarters

½ cup plain Greek yogurt

½ cup frozen unsweetened red raspberries

½ cup frozen blueberries

½ cup ice cubes

4 slices cucumber

Directions

1

Blend spinach, beet, yogurt, raspberries, blueberries, ice cubes, and cucumber together in a blender until smooth.

Nutritions

Per Serving: 256 calories; protein 9.8g; carbohydrates 33.5g; fat 10.9g; cholesterol 22.5mg; sodium 158.7mg.

CHAPTER 6: DESSERTS

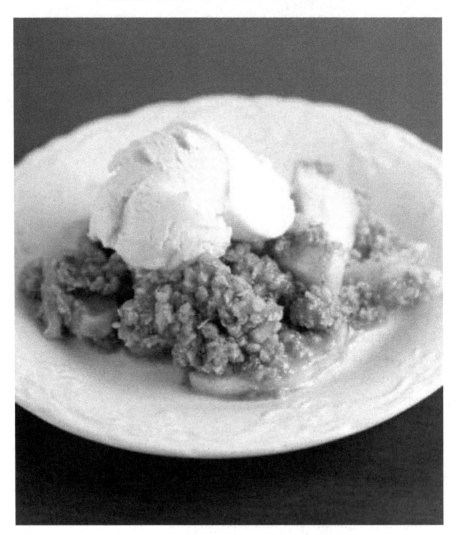

Apple Crisp

Prep:

20 mins

Cook:

35 mins

Additional:

45 mins

Total:

1 hr 40 mins

Servings:

4

Yield:

4 servings

Ingredients

4 apples - peeled, cored, and sliced

1 teaspoon vegetable oil

2 cups oats

1 teaspoon ground cinnamon

¼ cup butter

½ cup honey

1 cup brown sugar

Directions

1

Preheat oven to 350 degrees F.

2

Arrange apple slices in 9-inch circular glass pie plate.

3

Stir oats, brown sugar, and ground cinnamon together in a bowl.

4

Microwave butter in short 5-second increments until melted, about 20 seconds. Stir honey, melted butter, and oil into oat mixture; crumble over apples.

5

Bake in preheated oven until golden brown, about 35-40 minutes. Cool on a wire cooling rack, about 40-45 minutes.

Nutrition

Per Serving: 605 calories; protein 6g; carbohydrates 117.4g; fat 15.5g; cholesterol 30.5mg; sodium 97.4mg.

Red Sangria

Prep:

20 mins

Additional:

8 hrs

Total:

8 hrs 20 mins

Servings:

6

Yield:

6 servings

Ingredients

1 (750 milliliter) bottle Rioja red wine

¼ cup brandy

3 (1.5 fluid ounce) jiggers orange-flavored liqueur (such as Cointreau®)

1 large grapefruit

1 large lemon

1 clove pomander

1 large orange

ice cubes

2 limes, sliced

1 ½ cups lemon seltzer water

Directions

1

Pour Rioja into a large pitcher. Add brandy and orange liqueur. Cut orange, grapefruit, and lemon into wedges. Squeeze juice into the pitcher. Toss in fruit with rinds. Refrigerate until flavors combine, 8 hours to overnight.

2

Add pomander to the sangria several hours before serving.

3

Strain liquid into chilled glasses of ice. Top with a splash of seltzer. Garnish with lime slices.

Nutrition

Per Serving: 287 calories; protein 1.1g; carbohydrates 33.6g; fat 0.2g; sodium 7.5mg.

Almond Pudding

Prep:

10 mins

Cook:

20 mins

Additional:

3 hrs

Total:

3 hrs 30 mins

Servings:

8

Yield:

8 servings

Ingredients

2 cups almond meal

1 teaspoon instant espresso powder

¾ cup white sugar

1 teaspoon ground cinnamon

½ teaspoon ground cardamom

1 teaspoon vanilla extract

4 cups whole milk

Directions

1

Mix milk, almond meal, sugar, cinnamon, espresso powder, and cardamom in a large saucepan; bring to a simmer. Cook, stirring often, over low heat until slightly thickened, 20 minutes. Remove from heat and stir in vanilla extract. Chill in refrigerator until thickened, at least 3 hours.

Nutrition

Per Serving: 264 calories; protein 15.1g; carbohydrates 32.9g; fat 9.1g; cholesterol 12.2mg; sodium 50.9mg.

Chocolate Truffles

Prep:

30 mins

Additional:

1 hr 30 mins

Total:

2 hrs

Servings:

20

Yield:

20 servings

Ingredients

50 NILLA® waters

3 (.96 ounce) envelopes Swiss Miss® Simply Cocoa Dark Chocolate Hot Cocoa Mix

½ cup Reddi-wip® Original Dairy Whipped Topping

1 (3.25 ounce) cup Snack Pack® Chocolate Pudding

½ cup miniature marshmallows

1 cup premier white morsels

¼ teaspoon Coarse colored sugar

1 tablespoon Pure Wesson® Vegetable Oil

Directions

1

Line shallow baking pan with parchment paper; set aside. Place wafers and cocoa mix in food processor bowl; pulse wafers into fine crumbs. Add pudding and Reddi-wip; pulse until mixture comes together and forms a ball. Add marshmallows; pulse until marshmallows are cut into small pieces.

2

Roll wafer mixture into 1-inch balls; place on pan. Freeze 30 minutes or until set.

3

Place morsels and oil in small microwave-safe bowl. Microwave on HIGH 30 seconds; stir. Microwave on HIGH 30 seconds more or until softened; stir until mixture is melted completely. Roll a truffle in mixture until evenly coated. Remove with fork, letting excess drip off. Place on pan. Immediately sprinkle with some colored sugar, if desired. Repeat with remaining truffles. Refrigerate 1 hour or until firm. Store in airtight container in refrigerator.

Nutrition

Per Serving: 133 calories; protein 1.3g; carbohydrates 17.8g; fat 6.3g; cholesterol 4.6mg; sodium 74.1mg.

Biscotti

Prep:

15 mins

Cook:

25 mins

Total:

40 mins

Servings:

42

Yield:

3 to 4 dozen

Ingredients

½ cup vegetable oil

1 cup white sugar

3 eggs

1 tablespoon baking powder

1 tablespoon anise extract, or 3 drops anise oil

3 ¼ cups all-purpose flour

Directions

1

Preheat the oven to 375 degrees F. Grease cookie sheets or line with parchment paper.

2

In a medium bowl, beat together the oil, eggs, sugar and anise flavoring until well blended. Combine the flour and baking powder, stir into the egg mixture to form a heavy dough. Divide dough into two pieces. Form each piece into a roll as long as your cookie sheet. Place roll onto the prepared cookie sheet, and press down to 1/2 inch thickness.

3

Bake for 25 to 30 minutes in the preheated oven, until golden brown. Remove from the baking sheet to cool on a wire rack. When The cookies are cool enough to handle, slice each one crosswise into 1/2 inch slices. Place the slices cut side up back onto the baking sheet. Bake for an additional 6 to 9 minutes on each side. Slices should be lightly toasted.

Nutrition

Per Serving: 83 calories; protein 1.4g; carbohydrates 12.3g; fat 3.1g; cholesterol 13.3mg; sodium 40mg

White Peach-Lavender Compote

Prep:

5 mins

Cook:

5 mins

Additional:

1 hr

Total:

1 hr 10 mins

Servings:

4

Yield:

4 servings

Ingredients

1 ½ pounds white peaches, pitted and shopped
½ tablespoon lavender honey
5 sprigs lavender flowers

Directions

1

Combine peaches, honey, and lavender flowers in a microwave-safe bowl and cook for 5 minutes on high power. Discard lavender flowers.

2

Transfer peach mixture to a blender; blend until smooth. Cover with plastic wrap and refrigerate for 1 hour. Serve chilled.

Nutritions

Per Serving: 76 calories; protein 1.7g; carbohydrates 18.7g; fat 0.5g; sodium 1.2mg.

Cantucci Toscani

Servings:

36

Yield:

3 dozen (approx.)

Ingredients

4 cups all-purpose flour
2 cups white sugar
2 teaspoons baking powder
6 eggs
¼ cup hazelnut liqueur
2 teaspoons vanilla extract
2 teaspoons almond extract
2 cups hazelnuts - toasted, skinned and coarsely chopped

Directions

1

Mix dry **Ingredients** (except nuts) in a large bowl. Mix the eggs and liquids in a separate bowl. Add liquids to the dry **Ingredients** gradually, mixing until dough is stiff. Do not overmix. Stir in or work in the nuts.

2

Shape dough into two rectangles 3 inches wide, 15 inches long. Place on greased cookie sheet.

3

Bake for 20 minutes at 350 degrees F (175 degrees C). Remove baked rectangles from oven and let stand until cool to the touch.

4

Using sharp knife, slice rectangles crosswise into 3/4 inch slices. Place back on cookie sheet, sliced side down, and bake again for 15 minutes or until they are golden brown. Store in airtight container. These store well for weeks.

Nutritions
Per Serving: 160 calories; protein 3.6g; carbohydrates 23.9g; fat 5.5g; cholesterol 31mg; sodium 39.2mg.

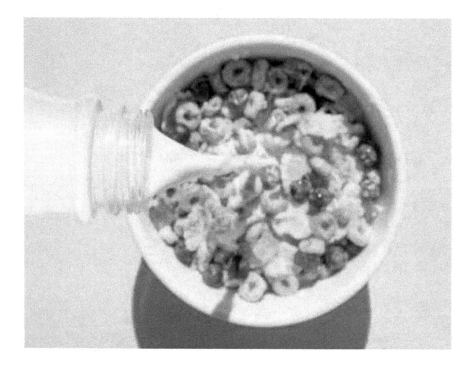

CPSIA information can be obtained
at www.ICGtesting.com
Printed in the USA
BVHW090319220621
610126BV00011B/2321

9 781803 303284